10 MINUTE BODYWEIGHT ROUTINES

HIGH PERFORMANCE BODYWEIGHT TRAINING WORKOUTS FOR STRENGTH AND CONDITIONING (NO GYM. NO SPECIAL EQUIPMENT REQUIRED.)

By Michael Martelli

Copyright © 2015

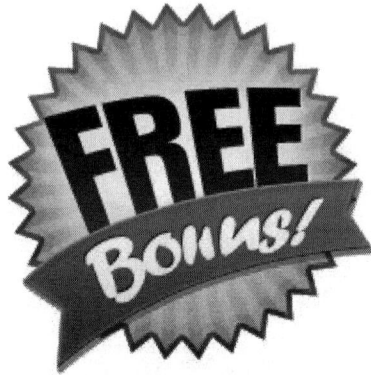

FREE BONUS GIFT:

The 30 Day Low Carb Diet Ketosis Plan

Thank you so much for purchasing this book!

As a thank you, and to get our relationship started right, I'd love to offer you're a **free** copy of "The 30 Day Low Car Diet Ketosis Plan."

This bonus picks up where this book leaves off and will help further guide you through an entire month of your weigh loss journey.

I am offering this because I think it's an excellent complement to this book, and because I want to see you succeed and reach your health goals.

Get your free ebook bonus right here.

INTRODUCTION

I want to thank you and congratulate you for choosing to download this book, "10 minute Bodyweight Routines."

It may come as quite a surprise to you that there are still thousands of muscle bound men and women that are convinced that the only way to develop their muscles is to spend hours at the gym pumping iron.

Little do they understand that there are other ways and these do not include hefty gym membership fees nor is there any equipment to be purchased!

Listen to me, all you need to do is pay attention and all you need is your body. The very best part of knowing about your body is when you finally realize that it can build itself, now that is what I call cool!

Why I Decided to Transform?

I was tired of being the only one in my group of friends without abdominals and I really wanted to get my body in the best shape possible. I wanted to get back my confidence again and look down and see a beautifully toned stomach. This wasn't going to be just a fitness transformation for me; it was a life transformation too. I had made up my mind that it was time to change and live a happy, healthy life.

How I Accomplished My Goals

At this time the majority of my friends were active, they swam, took aerobics or dance classes where as I was a mum of two small children, out of shape, overweight, tired and really fed up with what I had let myself become. I had a great support system however I had no a gym pass and very little nutrition knowledge, so I did 2-3 cardio sessions per day which included swimming, hiking, push-ups and sit-ups. I suppose the best way I could describe it was to compare it to watching Rocky train in terrain whilst every other member of the human race had the use of a gym.

I learned to diet through internet research and my girl friends that were immensely supportive. Yes I won't lie I had embarked on some of the toughest months ever, I stuck through it with sheer determination each and every day by looking at inspirational physiques and knowing that someday it would be me!

Training was what kept me on track

As I said earlier I didn't have the luxury of a gym pass or the money available to avail myself of one. Therefore I was left with bodyweight exercises and free-running cardio. Take it from me, don't let a gym be an excuse not to get in the best shape ever. Bodyweight exercises also opened my mind to exercising indoors and out in fact I could exercise wherever I was and there were no excuses as I didn't need a gym or any equipment in fact all I needed was me!

Whilst I found it a challenge when friends stated that they were just off to the gym and I would be lying if I didn't admit some days I found it a really battle to stay motivated, yet I knew that if I didn't keep working at this I would never get to where I am today.

My Future Fitness Plans

In the future, I would like to move things on a step and help others to develop their levels of fitness and show them how this can be achieved in a relatively short period of time with just dedication and a few minutes a day.

For those who are about to embark on a lifestyle change and develop their best body ever I would choose just two words: stay motivated!

Even when you simply cannot see it there is always light at the end of the tunnel. Don't worry if you have days where you fail disastrously as a winner will keep going even after failure. It is important that you are ready to dedicate just a little bit of time out of your day to give up what you are now for what you want to become in the future. Remember always that with hard work comes great success.

By reading this book you will gain a true insight into the huge benefits that bodyweight exercises can bring you. You will also see that there are no reasons for you not to undertake this type of exercise routine as you really can complete the exercises anywhere without any specialized equipment; you really do just need a little time and yourself!

I can honestly say that whilst I had off days where I missed exercising for one excuse or another however even taking this into account I found that results began to show after just two and a half months and over the past year I have lost two stone and whilst I am still working my way towards my goal, my body is certainly in far better shape.

No longer am I the one left sitting watching my children in the swimming pool because I am too embarrassed to don a costume. Yes there are still some lumps and bumps but I have had two children so what do you expect?

It is easy for me to tell you over and over again to take the initiative but you will only believe what I am saying by getting on with the bodyweight plan yourself.

Stop making excuses and give it a go, if it isn't for you then at least you can say you tried. Make today the beginning of the rest of your life, enjoy and very soon you will be strutting your stuff with an enviable body and be able to tell people when they ask truthfully that you don't spend hours in the gym just 10 – 15 minutes a day to stay in fabulous shape.

TABLE OF CONTENTS

LEGAL NOTES

Please note that the author strongly recommends that you consult with your physician or healthcare provider prior to beginning any type of exercise program.

When beginning any fitness regime you should be in good physical condition and be able to participate in the exercises freely with nothing to hamper your results.

The writer is not a licensed medical care provider and represents that they have no expertise in diagnosing, examining, or treating medical conditions of any kind, or in determining the effect of any specific exercise on a medical condition.

You must understand that when participating in any exercise or exercise program, there is the possibility of physical injury. If you engage in this exercise or exercise program, you agree that you do so at your own risk, are voluntarily participating in these activities, assume all risk of injury to yourself, and agree to release and discharge the writer or publisher from any and all claims or causes of action, known or unknown, arising out of negligence with regards to this publication or content included within.

Chapter 1 – What is Bodyweight Training?

Way before the introduction if exercise machines and equipment those who wanted to gain strength and muscle had to train simply by using their bodyweight. Although this concept originated because there was no alternatives it is a method of training still in use today due to its efficacy.

Bodyweight training alone has a long history and has been a consistent element use particularly by military organizations for hundreds of years. This is more than likely due to bodyweight training being inexpensive and the convenience of needing no specialized equipment and as such something that can be done anywhere.

Apart from the military uses, bodyweight exercises continue to be used in the athletic world and are also a main part in the majority of fat loss and muscle gain workouts available worldwide.

When we look at a complete program that uses weights as well, bodyweight training has some specific benefits, as well as bodyweight training being proven to be effective generally bodyweight exercises are profoundly different to the majority of weight bearing exercises even when the same muscles or movements are used.

WHY ARE THEY DIFFERENT?

Bodyweight exercises such as push – ups, lunges etc belong to a group of movements referred to as close kinetic chain exercises. These exercises are those where the hand or foot is fixed and does not move regardless of the rest of the body.

When these exercises are compared to exercises such as bench press, leg curls etc which belong to the group of movements referred to as open kinetic chain exercises. These exercises are performed without the hand or foot being fixed and allow movement with the rest of the body.

Generally if you move your body towards or away from an object the chain is closed whereas moving something towards to or away from your body the chain is open.

There is a huge difference between a person pulling themselves towards an object and pulling an object towards them when they are in a fixed position in terms of both muscular and neurological activation. Adding bodyweight closed kinetic chain exercises to your workout stimulates the nervous system in a completely different way than open kinetic chain exercises. There are some closed chain kinetic exercises considered to be superior as they require multiple muscle groups to coordinate in a movement.

COMBINING CLOSED AND OPEN KINETIC CHAIN EXERCISES

Although open chain kinetic exercises are probably more functional than any bodybuilding or strength training combining the two is always going to give you the best results.

Combining a variety of exercises exposes the nervous system to many types of stimuli and helps to increase the efficiency therefore a good combination of CKC exercises and OKC exercises will overtime increase both your strength and tone.

It should also be noted that due to no equipment being required you can easily move from one exercise to the next smoothly which not only saves you time but it is also a way to keep your rest periods short, your heart rate elevated and increase your metabolism.

Bodyweight training is not only effective on its own but by adding it to a program that includes weights will increase efficacy too.

Bodyweight training is the ideal choice for people of all ages regardless of their level of fitness.

CHAPTER 2 – THE SCIENCE BEHIND SHORT WORKOUTS AND HIIT

Being able to spend less time exercising yet still reaping real benefits could leave you thinking things are too good to be true. Long gone are the days of pounding the treadmill for 60 minutes straight as the philosophy of fitness has evolved with society.

The majority of us wants fast results and simply do not have the luxury of time to spend an hour but finding 10 – 15 minutes in our busy schedule is possible. Whilst you may be skeptical, there is a number of fitness findings that should make you think again.

FITNESS FINDINGS

Martin Gibala the physiologist at McMaster University, Ontario along with his colleagues published a study in 2006 that showed by that a 3 minute exercise sequence using a stationary bike and undertaking 30 seconds of furious pedaling followed by a short rest then repeating the sequence 5 times had the same results as 1.5 hours of prolonged bike riding.

Since this revelation ongoing studies have proved that just a few minutes of strenuous exercise can improve a person's aerobic fitness more quickly than lengthy moderate exercise.

Several other study and research have concluded that short bouts of exercise can yield better results than slow, steady workouts and it is from these findings that HIIT (high intensity interval training) evolved and is not the number one choice for many.

What is HIIT?

High intensity interval training involves intense bouts of exercise and low intensity exercise such as sprinting for 30 seconds then walking for a minute and so on.

Benefits of HIIT

There are a number of benefits offered by HIIT as well as this form of exercises offering serious fat burning, including:

-   Your oxygen uptake increases so your overall aerobic capacity increases faster than it would with low intensity endurance exercise.
-   The body can deal with the increase in lactic acid as your muscles increase.
-   Your muscles can deal with glucose and the glucose no longer goes to your fat stores.

HIIT workout

HIIT workouts are not suitable for beginners and should only be followed by those capable of completing a 30 minute cardio session working at 75 - 85% of their maximum heart rate. You could still do low intensity training and complete beginners should always wear a heart rate monitor.

For those considering HIIT it is vital that at least three minutes are dedicated to warming up and a further three minutes to cooling down as this will prevent any dizziness or feelings of nausea.

ONCE YOU BEGIN BODYWEIGHT TRAINING YOU WILL SOON REALIZE THAT A NUMBER OF WHAT ARE CONSIDERED BODYWEIGHT EXERCISES FORM THE BASIS OF MOST HIIT WORKOUTS.

CHAPTER 3 – BODYWEIGHT SPECIFICS

As you start out on your bodyweight journey you need to determine what your goals are, as without setting goals you will have no reason to work at something. These goals are most likely to center on the following:

- What is it that you want to do?
- Do you want to be bigger, stronger or a bit of both?
- What do you want to be good at?

Determining your goals should be easy and quite straightforward as generally people want strength, endurance, size, certain skills or a combination of these. It is also worth noting that strength will help with almost everything you are trying to improve, therefore if you have a combination of things it is worth focusing on your strength first.

With your goals determined the next step is to choose your goal exercises which are the skills you want to achieve. Due to the vast exercises incorporated in bodyweight fitness there is absolutely no way that you will be able to do everything although there is a lot of carryover in goals that are similar. It is advisable to choose up to 5 goal skills that you can begin working towards.

THE WAY BODYWEIGHT FITNESS WORKS

Bodyweight fitness does not consist of endless press ups or rounds of basic exercises. Bodyweight training is real resistant training.

Strength

In order to gain strength you should look to complete 3 – 5 sets, with 3 – 8 repetitions of heavy exercise which as much rest as you require between the sets. Your aim is to increase the amount of resistance between your workouts.

Muscle Size

To increase muscle size you should look to complete 3 sets, 8 – 12 repetitions of heavy exercise, resting for two minutes between sets.

Endurance

For endurance you should work the exercise/s you want to improve and do a lot of them!

The repetition ranges shown are fairly random and this is really down to your own personal choice and there is a lot of overlap. Three sets of 3 – 8 repetitions covers muscle growth whereas three sets with 8 – 12 repetitions will also cover strength. Beginners are advised to start with 3 sets and 5 – 8 repetitions.

Most importantly you need to learn how to increase the resistance of any given exercise and that is done by following progressions. A progression is a series of exercises from the same type/.group where each exercise is slightly more difficult than the previous one. You begin and work on the first exercise until you have built enough strength to be able to do the first exercise and the second exercise for a few repetitions. You then continue working on exercise number 2 until you are ready to work on the third exercise.

The following is a good practical example:

If you have chosen a pushup but you are unable to do a pushup, start by doing the pushup against the wall (vertical pushup) once you have mastered this move onto pushups on a raised surface such as a desk (incline pushups) and when you are competent at this you can move onto regular pushups.

The progression followed in this example would be:

Vertical pushup - incline pushups - regular pushups.

Be prepared as you will find that you cannot move up in terms of difficulty in every workout as the progression steps will be too hard. However to move up in difficulty you can also add repetitions. In most cases you will be capable of moving up once you can complete 3 x 10 of the current exercise.

BODYWEIGHT TRAINING

Muscle building with bodyweight training

It is possible to build muscle with bodyweight training and this is where your diet comes into play. Diet is

80% when it comes to how you look and in order to gain muscle (provided you are at your recommended weight) you will need to eat more. Training to gain muscle will see you doing a progression that you can do for 3 sets with 8 – 12 repetitions for each exercise and rest for no longer than one and a half minutes in between.

Strength work & Skill work

Skill work comprises of anything that requires a lot of practice in order for you to improve. Skill work does not have strength as the main element.

The handstand is a good example of skill work. Strength is needed for you to hold yourself up however balance is a huge element. Beginners do not have the strength to hold themselves up would mainly be improving their strength with a handstand and balance would not play a great part therefore for a beginner a handstand would be strength work. As the beginner gets stronger the handstand becomes all about balance as strength is no longer a significant element, this is when the beginners handstand becomes skill work.

Ideally you should separate skill and strength work. Your skill work should be relatively easy and not tiring so that you get the most from your time practicing. Skills would be practiced before your strength work and form part of your warm up, this also means that you will not be tired for your strength work. Use either a certain number of attempts or a preset amount of time to practice.

All exercises that require more strength that anything else are not skill work. This could mean moves such as the handstand or L-sits would fall under strength work, however this would only be to begin with. It is important to dedicate time to skill work if things such as the handstand are part of your end goal.

Equipment

You will need something to perform pull ups as these are vital to fix imbalances that the majority of people have. However this type of equipment can be a tree branch or stair well, it is also possible to use ropes, towels etc. These would be thrown over anything sturdy if it is not possible to hold onto the branch etc.

When completing inverted rows hanging under a sturdy table, tree etc can be used as equipment. Alternatively you could use a broom or other straight strong object placed across 2 chairs.

For dips you can use the backs of 2 chairs just remember to put heavy objects on the chairs if you think that they may fall over whilst you are using them.

The best place for you to execute L-sits is the floor.

You can even make your own equipment if you are a creative type all you need to be sure of is that it is safe.

Progressions

There are a number of free internet sources where you can glean information about the various forms of progressions in different exercises.

Leg work

There are not very many leg exercises when it comes to bodyweight training. It appears that squat and leg curl variations are all you have to work with, but these are adequate and have benefits for those wanting to work on their legs.

Further leg exercises are available using barbell training. Calf raises have not been included as these are not difficult and offer no progressions without adding weight.

Therefore we will concentrate on the multiple ways that you can include squats and deadlifts into your bodyweight training. The following are the two most solid options:

- Make squats part of every workout and add deadlifts once a week at the end of your workout.
- Squats incorporated into two of your workouts and deadlifts in the other workout as your leg exercises.

The recommended exercise requirement for squats is 3 sets of 5 repetitions and for deadlifts 1 set of 5 repetitions. It is advisable to do 1 – 3 sets of deadlifts and squats using a light weight as a warm up prior to continuing with squats and deadlifts.

Development

One your progress slows or plateaus in your beginner routine, it is probably time for you to switch to an intermediate routine. The initial changes deal with the weekly frequency and you will be completing specific exercise, allowing more time for recovery whilst introducing deloads.

In order to implement this you need to:

1) Choose a set and repetition goal

This needs to be based on whether you want strength, muscle size or endurance along with different amounts of repetitions. The recommendation for a beginner is still 5 – 8 repetitions whilst the 3 – 5 repetition is ideal for the more difficult exercises with the set remaining the same in the range of 3 – 5.

2) Pick a template either from those below or one that you have researched yourself

- Full body, 2 day – 2 workouts both incorporating 1 x push, 1 x matching pull, 1 x leg exercise plus 1 x core exercise.
- Push/pull split – 2 workouts both incorporating 2 – 3 x push exercises and 1 x leg exercises. The other will contain 2 – 3 x pull exercises plus 1 x leg extensions.

- Push/pull/leg splits – 3 workouts one incorporating 2 – 3 x push exercises and support hold work, The final workout contains 2 – 3 leg exercises and core work

- Volume/light/heavy – 3 workouts with various repetitions and progressions. Each workout contains 1 x push, 1 x pull, 1 x leg and 1 x core exercises. The volume workout is executed with higher repetitions which are typically 10 – 12 range. The light workout is done using easier progressions with medium repetitions typically in the 5 – 8 range. The heavy workout is completed using your top progression for fewer repetitions typically in the range of 3 – 5.

3) Choose your workout time

You workout routine should fit into your schedule and the following are both ways in which you can achieve this:

- 3 days a week with a rest day in between. This is the standard Monday/Wednesday/Friday layout and you alternate through each workout

- 2 days on,1 day off is the layout that sees you performing two workouts back to back followed by a rest day. This is the best time schedule for the split templates in point 2 above, as there is less overlap between the days.

4) Choose certain exercises to fill your template

It is advisable to test your performance on a given exercise to be included in your own routine. Start with a warm up and test the movements in all the progressions that you plan to use. You should pick an exercise where you are capable of completing the amount of repetitions is the correct foundations for good form. If you find that you cannot complete the repetitions for your goal you should choose easier progressions and vice versa if you can manage even more repetitions.

5) Organize your exercises

Begin with the exercise that you most want to improve. Perform 3 – 5 sets of this exercise resting for as long as you feel is necessary before you move onto the second most important of your exercises. Bear in mind if you have included both pushes and pulls these should be ideally rotated.

6) Add skill before strength

Skill work is sport specific and helps you to reach your goals. Skill work is none or low fatigue and is more time limited. Anything requiring more practice that effort should be seen as skill work. The standard recommendation when looking at skill work is to practice the exercise for an allocated amount of time including your rest. Focus on resting and make any attempts good ones with minimal fatigue.

Handstands and L sits fall into basic skills and have real benefits worth working on. Balance and agility make an excellent addition to any intermediate level. Exercises such as yoga tree poses, single legged calf raises etc can all help to build these attributes.

Remember anything that requires more strength that anything else is not considered as skill work.

7) Warm up

The aim of a warm up is to warm your entire body and be able to perform your exercises through a complete range of motions whilst using muscles to an extent that they are not usually used. If you have any mobility issues which prevent you from performing the exercises now is the time for these to be addressed. Finish your warm up with exercises that will get your blood flowing.

8) Conditioning

Although optional, conditioning is recommended and includes exercises such as running, cycling, jumping rope etc. Conditioning can either be performed on days when you are not strength training or added to the end of your workout.

9) Time to go

Have fun as you begin your training!

Routines that consist of warm up, skill work, strength work, a few exercises and flexibility work can take a lot of time and not everyone has the luxury of time.

The best way to save time is to complete your mobility and flexibility work on your days off. These elements are not taxing and could even help your recovery.

The second concerns strength work. If you are already doing mobility on your days off and you're strengthening routine still takes too long you might want to consider pairing your exercises. For example if you normally workout with pushups and rows with a 3 minute rest between sets these can easily be paired by completing a set of pushups, rest for 1.5 minutes and do a set of rows before taking another 1.5 minute break. This works because the pairing doesn't use that many overlapping muscles so the rowing doesn't have a big impact on the rest you are taking from the pushups and vice versa.

If you still find that you haven't got enough time, consider dropping some of the exercises or splitting the volume over different workout days.

CHAPTER 4 – ALL YOU NEED IS YOUR BODY

Thinking that the only way to get the body you want means going to the gym twice a day would scare even the most dedicated person. The good news is that this book can show you that to take control of your health and achieve great things is possible in less time than you could ever imagine.

Not only is there no need to spend hour upon hour in the gym you actually don't need to go to the gym at all!

Spending hours in the gym is the old way and whilst it is effective it really is not a necessity. Looking at modern day training it is necessary to look at metabolic resistance training (MRT).

The most important things to take onboard about MRT are as follows:

- Metabolic resistance training essentially refer to fast paced circuits where your aim is to move from one exercise to the next with very little rest in between.
- Metabolic resistance training is proven to be one of the most effective training for weight loss.

- Metabolic resistance training can be done using any kind of equipment or nothing at all in just 10 – 15 minutes.

Point 3 above is what you should focus on immediately and these are the exercises that can be completed in just 10 minutes with no need for equipment. Now look at point 2 above and this tells you that these workouts have been proven to be one of the most effective ways to lose weight, It is also proven that this workout can be done effectively in 10 – 15 minutes with no equipment and still be one of the most effective ways of burning fat and getting in shape.

Yes, it does sound too good to be true and equally hard to believe but effective bodyweight training can be merely 1% of your day.

You may still be skeptical and find it really hard to comprehend that you can get a great workout with just your bodyweight, and a workout that takes just 10 minutes and can be done by anyone, anywhere.

The time is right to take the next step and embark on taking control and dedicate 10 minutes most days to get the body that you have only ever dreamed about.

CHAPTER 5 – COMPONENTS OF AN EXERCISE PROGRAM

There are six components if a workout routine and whilst each component may be shown by a different name, the components themselves are exactly the same.

These components are:

1) Warm up
2) Stretching
3) Cardio training
4) Muscular training
5) Cool down
6) Stretching

It is important that you realize that every component has to be completed. There are far too many people that do not perform each of the above steps for whatever reason and by doing so they dramatically increase their chance of injury. Many people either don't stretch or do so only briefly and this results in them being forced to stop exercising.

1) Warm up

Your warm up should be a low rhythmic aerobic exercise that involves all the major muscle groups such as your legs. The warm up is preparation if your body for more intensive exercise. The low intensity warm up should last for at least five minutes and must be completed first before anything else.

2) Stretching

This type of stretching is very low intensity and is designed to comfortably stretch certain muscle groups. Each stretch pose should be held for 20 – 30 seconds and ideally you should stretch out your muscles every day.

3) Cardio training

The purpose of cardio training is to complete a form of aerobic exercises such as jogging, stair climbing etc and to 80% of your maximum heart rate.

You can calculate your heart rate by taking your heart rate and taking off your age. Therefore if you heat rate is 210 and you are 30 years old: 210 – 30 = 180. To work out at 80% your heart rate would need to be 154. Cardio training also sees you burning fat from 65% of your heart rate onwards therefore once your heart rate reaches 127 you are beginning to burn the fat.

Cardio training needs to be completed 3 times a week for about half an hour per session. It is worth considering your daily housework chores as these will easily fit into this meaning there may be no need for you to do anything else as a separate activity.

4) Muscle training

Muscle training can be done with or without weight machines and whilst the activity requires the use of free weights these can easily be objects around your home. Muscle training should be undertaken for the minimum of 20 minutes, 2 – 3 times a week.

5) Cool down

The cool down is vital and is low intensity, rhythmic aerobic exercises designed to help your body return to its pre exercise state. Your cool down should follow your training exercises and last for no less than three minutes.

6) Stretching

The final set of stretches is simply to stretch out the muscle groups to avoid them from getting stiff and sore. Whenever you undertake any form of bodyweight training the emphasis is strongly on quality as opposed to quantity.

GETTING TOO BIG

Many people that start exercising believe that their muscles may get too big for what they are trying to achieve, however this is highly unlikely as it takes time, and total dedication to obtain body builders style mass. In order to look this way you would have to be exercising 6 days a week for a minimum of 4 hours a day intensely training your muscles.

CHAPTER 6 – BODYWEIGHT WORKOUT FOR BEGINNERS

You have decided that you want to get in shape; however you don't want the expense of gym membership. That's fine because a lot of the time gyms are full of either ultra serious beings or those who haven't got a clue!

As luck would have it you can burn fat, build muscle and get a great workout just by using your own bodyweight. By learning why cardio is one of the least efficient way of burning calories and you will see how easy it is to get a lot done in a very small space of time. Completing lots of bodyweight circuits where one exercise follows on from another without stopping not only will you build muscle but you are performing a good cardio workout too.

WHY BODYWEIGHT CIRCUITS ARE SO GOOD

Every exercise that is part of the bodyweight circuit uses multiple groups of muscle, gets your heart pumping and burns a huge amount of calories. Circuit weight training burns far more calories that interval training which burns far more calories than steady cardio. For those trying to lose weight, spending hours of your time doing cardio, i.e. on a treadmill will really not be worth your time.

BASIC BODYWEIGHT ROUTINE/CIRCUIT

The following beginners bodyweight routine can be completed anywhere. It is really important particularly for those who have done little or no exercise to check with their doctor or health care provider before proceeding.

In this routine each exercise follows on without any rest breaks (provided that you are capable of doing so). Once you have completed the circuit you start all over again. If you find at the end of this 2nd circuit that you can continue for a 3rd then go for it!

Due to the exercises being one after another it is inevitable that you will get tired, and it is far better to stop at this point than to do the exercise incorrectly and risk injury. If you find that you cannot complete 3 circuits without stopping it is not a bad thing as it gives you something to progress towards.

The most important thing before you start is to warm up. This is vital and must never be forgotten as it gets your muscles warm and your heart rate pumping. Forget this step and you asking for an injury. If you are lacking time cut your workout short, not the warm up.

For your warm up you can run on the spot, pedal on a bike, skip etc. The aim is to warm your body up and elevate your heart rate. Once warmed up you are ready to begin.

Beginner's bodyweight routine

20 x bodyweight squats
10 x push ups
20 x walking lunges
10 x dumbbell rows
15 second plank
30 x Jumping jacks

To begin if you have trouble with the bodyweight squats or lunges use your hand to support and keep you balanced. When completing the bodyweight squats think of it as sitting back in a chair and then standing immediately without leaning forwards. When completing the lunges keep looking straight ahead and keep your upper body completely vertical. When doing the dumbbells use whatever object that is heavy enough for you, make sure it is challenging to lift 10 times in a row.

Once you have completed the workout it is important to stretch as all of your muscles will have contracted and need to be stretched back out so that they can repair.

You should aim to do this workout 2 – 3 times a week but not on consecutive days because you don't build muscle whilst exercising, it is built by resting. As you muscles need time also to repair your exercise plan for a week may look as follows:

Day 1 – Strength training
Day 2 – Bodyweight routine

Day 3 – Strength training
Day 4 - Bodyweight routine
Day 5 – Cardio workout
Day 6 - Bodyweight routine
Day 7 – Rest

Along with your bodyweight routine it is really important that you eat properly. If you have a really good exercise schedule but fill your face with junk you won't get anywhere. Remember from earlier that your diet is 80% of your success or failure.

Chapter 7 – Form an exercise routine with just bodyweight exercises

Whether you can't get to the gym, are traveling for work, don't have the money or access to the equipment, or the understanding on how to add bodyweight exercises into your daily routine are a great choice for those who live a healthy and active lifestyle.

There are endless amounts of exercises that don't require a gym setting, also all manner of combinations you can choose in order to get into the habit of taking regular exercise.

Again before you begin you need to have a goal in mind such as:

1) If your goal is fat loss, you need to focus on your diet along with the reasons why you eat what you do.
2) If you goal is to increase your strength, making use of additional weight in a variety of exercises may prove the fastest route.
3) If your goal is athletic performance, your focus will be on recovery and enhanced rate of force production.

As you can see none of these actions alone will get you to your goal fastest. There is no doubt that your bodyweight exercises will enhance however to accelerate towards your goal will see you using a combination of methods.

Regardless of your goal, bodyweight exercises will get you there provided that you vary your movements to prevent overuse of any single movement pattern, and also relieve boredom and or deviation from your path to goal.

Due to fat loss requiring a nutritional focus and not something covered with this book and athletic performance being very specific and dependant on the sport, I will continue with a goal of increasing strength and using your bodyweight to complete these feats from your first push up right through to performing your first ever triple clap push up!

BUILDING YOUR ROUTINE

When constructing your routine it is important to keep the following at the forefront of your mind:

1) Horizontal pushing
2) Horizontal pulling
3) Vertical pulling
4) Vertical pushing
5) Quad domination
6) Hip hinge
7) Single leg quad
8) Single hip hinge
9) Anti – extension
10) Anti – rotation

11) Anti – flexion
12) Combination movements – lateral and multi – planar movements

Amongst these there are also opportunities to do exercises that enhance the stretch, improve your neural drive for improvements in jumping etc.

Now this information is collated you are ready to start making your own unique bodyweight routine.

THE STEPS

1) Step 1 – Warm up

You warm up must come before anything else for the following reasons:

- Muscles that surround other joints may have been underactive
- Improve neural drive towards patterns of movement and can help to increase the performance if the actual exercises
- Completing a variety of exercises may help your movement patterns to be maintained even when they are not the focus

2) Step 2 – Exercise programs

Circuit A – perform three times for your own personal designated duration.

- Hip hinge – this is a vertical jump, pause on landing

- Anti – rotation – complete the side plank
- Vertical pushing – yoga style push up
- Single leg quad – squat split
- Vertical pulling – chin ups provided that you have the right equipment at your disposal

Circuit B – perform three times for your own personal designated duration.

- Dominant quad – bodyweight squat to chair with your hands behind your head
- Anti – extension – front plank
- Horizontal pulling – Prone Ts
- Single leg hip hinge – single leg lift and reach
- Horizontal pushing – push up

3) Step 3 – After workout stretching

The after workout stretching really is self explanatory. Now that you have a good base you can start to appreciate that as long as you apply all of the principles you can easily create an effective exercise program. One that will not only make you sweat, but gets your heart racing and also keeps you in the right mindset.

CHAPTER 8 – REASONS TO START BODYWEIGHT TRAINING TODAY

Getting fit does not need to be a complicated process and simple bodyweight exercises can be the perfect choice for advancing strength building muscle, boosting cardio fitness and burning fat. For those who are still not convinced, the following points may change your mind and make you realize why bodyweight exercises should be a major element of your workout routine.

1) Super efficient workouts

Provided your aspiration is not to look like a body building muscle bound champion the days of 2 hour workouts are well and truly a thing of the past. Studies and research all point towards high output bodyweight exercises bringing fantastic fitness results in very short periods of time. With no equipment, bodyweight exercises make it easy to move from one exercise to the next effortlessly. Plus the short rest periods means that the heart rate is quickened and you burn serious calories.

2) Combination training (cardio and strength)

Regardless of time constraints there is no reason why you cannot do a quick cardio and strength workout such as jumping jacks between your strength exercises as these will keep your heart pumping whilst also encouraging strength and muscle development.

3) Speedy fat burn

If you are looking to lose a few pounds, just sparing a few minutes with bodyweight training and you can. This is because bodyweight training has a major impact on your metabolism. Whether you believe it or not, try it and see the results.

4) Enjoyable by all

Bodyweight exercises are ideal as they can be tailored to challenge all levels of fitness. Simply by adding some extra repetitions or performing the exercises faster or really slow are all ways that can make even the simplest exercises challenging. Your progress is easy to measure as bodyweight exercises offer a number of ways to do more with every workout.

5) Core strength

Your core covers far more than just the abdominals. There are at least 29 muscles that make up the human core and there are lots of simple bodyweight movements can be used to engage them all.

6) More flexibility

Bodyweight training for strength and flexibility can easily go hand in hand. Undertaking complete bodyweight exercises by using a full range of motion.

Making sure that your joints are moving freely can assist with your posture and may even reduce the chance of injury from exercise. Yoga which is a bodyweight workout choice chosen by many as it is a great way to improve strength and flexibility.

7) Convenience

The chances are if you were to ask people why they don't exercise their answer would be "no time" or because they find exercise an inconvenience. Bodyweight exercises eliminate a lot of the obstacles and allow anyone to work out wherever they may be. No equipment exercise can be a great stress reliever for those who work at home or those that work away can easily make their bodyweight routine their hotel room workout. The essence behind the convenience really ensures there are no credible excuses!

8) Balance

As bodyweight exercises use no weights, there are other ways that you can increase the resistance. Functional exercises like the bodyweight squat can improve balance through increased body awareness.

9) No more boredom

It is far too easy to end up in a rut with regards to workouts. This is where and why bodyweight exercises are refreshing, as there are a number of variations to relieve boredom, and also break through any plateau you may find yourself in.

10) Making fitness fun

Exercising indoors is not to everyone's liking, therefore another plus of bodyweight exercises is they can be performed indoors or out, on your own or with a group of friends. You can also inject a little silliness making for even more fun.

11) Saving money

Joining a gym can be expensive but bodyweight training costs absolutely nothing. It is for this reason that bodyweight routines are enjoying a new lease of life with many followers. Additionally there are some excellent outdoor locations that are popping up and offer an amazing space for you to complete your free bodyweight workout.

12) Preventing injury

Injury is one of the main reasons that people stop exercising therefore preventing aches and pains should be a major priority. Bodyweight exercises in general are safe for all regardless of age, experience or fitness level.

Finally it is only fitting to mention the excellent results that can be achieved by doing bodyweight exercises. These results are mainly thanks to the compound movements which mean numerous joints and muscles are used together for each move. The results are further amplified because of the core strength they develop. Bodyweight training provides improved core strength throughout the entire body.

There is no one fits all when it comes to exercising, but bodyweight exercises offer many benefits that other forms of resistance can't. The huge popularity of boot camp style fitness and mobile fitness apps suggest people like the way they feel and the shape that they can achieve working out without weights.

If you are new to resistance training, don't panic and always remember the first rule and most important is to make sure you warm up properly.

CHAPTER 9 – WEIGHT TRAINING COMPARED TO BODYWEIGHT EXERCISES?

It is amazing how different the effects of weight training are compared to bodyweight training. But if we generalize and assume that your goals are safety, muscle size and strength then the results would be as follows:

- Muscle size and strength – weights
- Safety – bodyweight training

Weights will win over bodybuilding if you are talking about muscle size and strength. The very best bodybuilding builders achieve their muscle size through intensive weight training.

Regarding strength we will assume you mean strength as it's understood most commonly, the ability to move an object or mass. If you were to add a time component then you are talking about power. In both of these examples your body weight can be included as an object of mass. Therefore in both respects weights are far superior to bodyweight training simply because they allow for greater loads to be worked on.

Bodyweight training doesn't allow the way to replicate the ability to squat, bench, dead lift etc heavy weight.

The limit bodyweight training has is that you are stuck with a weight that doesn't change as in your bodyweight. When using weights you can continuously increase the weight in order to make you stronger.

Bodyweight training definition has its place when looking at an overall fitness regime. When embarking on bodyweight training, the risk of injury is greatly reduced and therefore it is much easier to incorporate bodyweight training in an intense anaerobic exercise.

Bodyweight training also teaches you to move your body more efficiently and with greater endurance. The majority of training regimes for functional strength also include a mix of bodyweight and weight training.

Bodyweight exercises and weight training are both effective in fitness training, in fact a good plan could use both to a varying degree. It doesn't matter what training plan you are following, you will eventually reach a plateau and my suggestion would be to change the training repetitions and sets for each exercise.

Bodyweight exercises focus more on strength due to the higher repetitions that are involved. Paying attention to appropriate food and enough regeneration with your bodyweight will not be enough on its own. To see further progress both muscular and strength wise you need to carry put lifting, pushing and also pulling weight. Failure to do so will find that your plan stagnates. Choose your exercises wisely and look to those that use multiple muscles and free weights.

Body weight exercises will win any day if real strength and fitness is your goal and this is because of how the muscles cooperate more naturally rather than the way they move when using weights. The so-called multi-joint exercises which see many muscle groups working together directly and indirectly will help to release the growth hormones and develop unparalleled strength.

For some inspiration in this department all we need to look at is male gymnasts, muscular but also with useful strength.

As well as all of this, use static training every now and then and with the mentioned exercises you are going to get fast results

CHAPTER 10 – BODYWEIGHT FAQS

In this chapter we will look at some of the frequently asked questions in order to enhance your workout and be sure that you are performing the right routine to achieve your specifics.

Qu1: What routine should I do?

For those with goals that have non-specific, strength based or are looking to grow muscle and lose fat then a traditional bodyweight routine is all that you will need. Be sure to remember that diet is a very important factor if you are looking to build muscle and lose fat

Qu2: I can't do the recommended routine as I have nowhere to do pull ups!

There are no excuses for this one. There are no alternatives to pull ups and they are really very important. Either buy a pull up bar or find a tree, staircase with some space underneath it, honestly the options really are limitless.

Qu3: I can't complete the recommended routine because I have nowhere to do rows!

It is quite easy to complete rows under a table or you can put a raised object in front of you. A stick balanced across two chairs may work equally as well or try hanging something from your pull up bar. Just be creative as there are many ideas and no excuses.

Qu4: I cannot complete my routine because I have nowhere to dip!

Anywhere the makes a 90° angle is suitable, as are the backs of two sturdy chairs or two boxes placed next to each other. Use your imagination and you will soon find that there are no excuses.

Qu5: Can I train every day?

The answer to this is dependent on your program. If you're training for muscle mass or strength it is important to know that you get stronger and bigger whilst you rest because of the super compensation effect. Training daily the strength/muscle mass is possible however this is a more advanced technique and should be programmed correctly, therefore if you need to ask this question it is most likely that this type of training is not for you.

Qu6: What can I do on my day on my off days?

If you are following a strength program like the beginner routine, you need to rest and your off days are in order for your body to recover and get stronger. This doesn't mean you have to you sit on your bum all day, you can still do a none taxing workout like going for a run or messing around in the park. For more specific bodyweight training you can do skill work such as handstands as these will help you improve your regular workouts.

Qu7: Should I complete all sets before I move on to the next?

If you are following a recommended routine then you should complete it as it is written. This means completing each exercise before moving onto the next pair. However if you are particularly looking for strength and weight loss or muscle mass then you should do all sets of one exercise before moving on to the next.

Qu8: Can I split my routine up over the day?

This isn't a problem for strength, although it will mean warming up every time you start a new block. If you are looking for muscle mass you may lose some stimulus for muscle growth however if you cannot fit your routine in any other way this is what you will have to do.

Qu9: How can I combine cardio with bodyweight training?

If you are running/swimming/rowing etc casually it will be fine for you to undertake these on your off days. The typical layout is to do cardio on off days exclusively, so that you have one true rest day per week however another way with more rests could be as follows:

Monday - bodyweight training and cardio
Tuesday - rest
Wednesday - bodyweight training and cardio
Thursday - rest
Friday - bodyweight training
Saturday - cardio
Sunday - rest

As you will see from this schedule you get a couple more rest days per week which will allow you to recover better. Generally cardio should be done after strength training and not before.

Qu10: What results can I expect using bodyweight training?

Providing that your diet and training are done correctly you can expect to gain muscle, lose fat and get stronger. You can build a nice body with bodyweight training.

Qu 11: How soon will I see results?

If you are following a good routine will see progress in the exercises in about 2 to 3 workouts. If your diet is in check you will certainly start to notice physical changes from about six weeks, but be prepared for it to take 12 weeks plus for your changes to be noticed by others.

Qu 12: I'm sore and I am not sure this is working, should I work out?

Soreness means very little however if you get to a stage where you can't move a body part then you should seek medical advice immediately.

Made in the USA
Middletown, DE
13 October 2015